Copyright ©

Legal & Disclaimer

The information contained in this book and its contents is not designed to replace or take the place of any form of medical or professional advice; and is not meant to replace the need for independent medical, financial, legal or other professional advice or services, as may be required. The content and information in this book have been provided for educational and entertainment purposes only.

You agree that by continuing to read this book, where appropriate and/or necessary, you shall consult a professional (including but not limited to your doctor, attorney, or financial advisor or such other advisor as needed) before using any of the suggested remedies, techniques, or information in this book.

TABLE OF CONTENTS

INTRODUCTION

The Dukan diet is a high protein, low carbohydrate eating plan designed by Pierre Dukan, a former French physician and self-proclaimed nutritionist.

Also called the Dukan method, this diet is based on how hunter-gatherers may have eaten.

The diet includes 100 foods, and all are either proteins or vegetables. A person can eat as much as they like, as long as they only eat those 100 foods.

The Dukan diet may contribute to weight loss, but research has linked it to possible health complications, including kidney disease and liver disease. Also, it may not provide the full range of nutrients the body needs.

PART ONE: THE DUKAN DIET OVERVIEW

What is the Dukan diet?

The Dukan diet is based on the theory that eating a lot of protein can help people lose weight. This is because:
• lean, high protein foods tend to be lower in calories
• eating protein can help people feel full
• digesting protein uses more energy, so the body burns a few more calories
Restricting carbs and fats induces a starvation-like state, which forces the body to use fat stores for energy, similar to the Atkin's diet.

The history of Dukan

Dubbed "the French medical solution to permanent weight loss", the Dukan diet is the ultimate in prescriptive eating, with just 72 foods to choose from in the first phase. Carbs are the enemy, even if they come dressed as fruit and veg.

Pierre Dukan's high-protein, low-carb plan was first published in France in 2000 under the name 'Je ne sais pas maigrir' (I don't know how to lose weight). It wasn't until 2010 that the Dukan movement reached the UK, rebranded as the Dukan diet. Despite being the new kid on an already very carb-free block, Dukan carved a gap in the jostling miracle weight loss market with a little help from some fairly well known fans. Kate Middleton, in the run up to her Royal wedding, reportedly dropped two dress sizes following Dukan's method.

Pierre Dukan began his medical career specialising in neurology but allegedly switched to nutrition after recommending a high-protein diet to a friend desperate to lose weight. So impressed with his friend's rapid reduction in size, Dukan embarked on developing and researching the diet that would eventually make him a household name. To date, the Dukan diet book has sold more than eight million copies worldwide and has been translated into 14 different languages.

Not without controversy, Dukan's weight loss plan has come under criticism from health professionals, many believing that the diet promotes an unbalanced way of eating. In recent years, Pierre Dukan's controversial claims have also brought unwanted attention upon the Dukan brand.

The original diet

The original Dukan diet is similar to a ketogenic diet as both emphasise the consumption of fat and protein but omit carbohydrates. The body will turn to glycogen stores (carbohydrates) for energy first if supplies are plentiful. Ketogenic diets essentially force the body to switch from burning carbohydrates for energy to burning fat. This often has the desirable effect of weight loss, though high levels of ketones in the body can be problematic and may lead to a state known as ketosis.

Phases

There are four phases in the Dukan diet:

1. Attack phase.

This first stage lasts between five-ten days and promises immediate results. Dieters have 72 high-protein foods to choose from, with absolutely no carbohydrates allowed.

2. Cruise phase.

While pure protein days are still encouraged, carbohydrates are slowly reintroduced in the form of 28 pre-approved vegetables. Dukanites stay in this stage until they have reached their 'goal weight'.

3. Consolidation phase

Previously forbidden foods such as fruit and dairy are gradually reintroduced. Followers are even granted two 'celebration meals' a week where they are allowed to eat almost anything they like (some restrictions still apply).

4. Stabilisation phase

If you've managed to reintroduce carbohydrates back into your life without putting weight back on, you're allowed to smugly step into stage 4 and unlock the 'rules for life'.

How long people stay on the diet depends on their current weight, fitness and desired goal weight.

The Dukan Diet 2

Since the development of the original Dukan diet, a second programme has been formulated which in essence reflects the original consolidation phase. Dukan 2 involves seven steps – each step represents the dietary inclusion of a food group. Steps one and two involve eating unlimited quantities of 100 allowed foods, which include natural proteins (step one) and vegetables (step two). Subsequent steps involve the graduated addition of fruit, breads, cheese and other starches, such as pasta.

Dukan Diet Attack Phase

The Attack phase is the first step of the Dukan Diet. It is also known as the Pure Protein (PP) phase. The sudden change in your eating habits triggers a fast and encouraging weight loss, which works to motivate you for the rest of your diet.

The Dukan Diet Attack phase: short, quick, and successful weight loss

 The duration of the Dukan Diet Attack phase depends on your age, the weight you need to lose, and the number of diets you have done in the past. The Dukan Diet Attack phase usually lasts from 2 to 5 days, here are some guidelines:

• Less than 10 lbs. to lose: 1 or 2 days
• From 15 to 30 lbs. to lose: 3 to 5 days

• More than 40 lbs. to lose: after consulting with your physician, this phase can last up to 7 days.

Ketosis: eat unlimited Pure Protein foods to avoid hunger and cravings.

Only NATURAL Pure Protein foods are allowed on the Attack phase: 68 animal proteins, in unlimited quantity. Some studies have proven that proteins produce a satiating effect.* The protein intake in the Dukan Diet Attack phase increases the speed of weight loss while flushing out the excess water from your body. The digestion of protein produces ketones which are eliminated in your urine. This is why it is imperative that you drink 6 to 8 cups of water a day. Oat bran will provide some carbs and daily fiber that bind to calories from the food consumed and limit their absorption.

Physical activity will optimize weight loss in the Dukan Diet Attack phase

Start exercising gradually during the Attack phase. Take advantage of the fat burning effect of exercise – particularly in the morning. No matter your fitness level, walking is an activity that anyone can do. It is natural, costs nothing, and has many benefits.

Dukan Diet Cruise Phase

The Cruise phase is the second phase of the Dukan Diet. It reintroduces vegetables with Proteins and Vegetables (PV) days and establishes the 100 unlimited allowed foods as a base. The goal of the Dukan Diet

Cruise phase is steady weight loss until you reach your True Weight.

Dukan Diet Cruise phase – steady weight loss to achieve your True Weight

Weight loss in the Cruise phase is gradual - on average, 1 lb. every 3 days. The desired effect is to get rid of body fat while maintaining lean body mass.

100 unlimited allowed foods

In addition to the 68 allowed proteins in the Attack phase and on PP days, you can add 32 non-starchy vegetables on PV days while on the Cruise phase.

The 100 allowed foods list contains foods that will supply you with vitamins, minerals, and fiber, thanks to their nutritional diversity. These foods make Dukan Cooking easy.

Alternating rhythms suited to your lifestyle

Alternation is always made up of the exact same number of Pure Protein (PP) and Proteins and Vegetables (PV) days. For example: 1/1 means 1 day of Protein and Vegetables followed with 1 day of Pure Protein and so on. If you are stagnating, you can use a higher alternation such as 2/2, 3/3, 4/4 or 5/5. The 5/5 is especially recommended for people who have a lot of weight to lose.

Physical activity prescription

On the Dukan Diet Cruise phase, 30 minutes of brisk walking will help maximize your weight loss.

DUKAN DIET CONSOLIDATION PHASE

The Consolidation phase is the third phase of the Dukan Diet. It marks the end of the weight loss phases after the Cruise phase, and retains the base of Proteins and Vegetables, plus a gradual reintroduction of starchier foods. The objective of the Dukan Diet Consolidation phase is to preserve and maintain your True Weightreached at the end of the Cruise phase.

Dukan Diet Consolidation phase

 This third phase of the Dukan Diet marks the transition between the strict food list and spontaneity. The Consolidation phase lasts 10 days for every pound lost, and corresponds to the time during which your body is still vulnerable to rebound weight gain. Completion of the phase will ensure that you will maintain your weight loss.

The Nutritional Stairs: the reintroduction of fun foods in limited amounts.

The seven steps of the Nutritional Stairs clearly show how the Dukan Diet Consolidation phase will become your new healthy eating plan and, step by step, will become a habit for life.

BASE: the 1st and 2nd steps are represented by the unlimited 100 allowed foods(Proteins and Vegetables), plus 1 serving of lamb and roast pork weekly. You are now allowed to use uncured cooked ham, and are not limited to extra lean.

Add the following foods to this base in ascending order:

Additions in the first half of Consolidation

• A serving of fruit every day*

• 2 slices of whole grain bread per day

- 1.5 ounces of hard rind cheese
- 1 serving (cooked cup) of starchy foods every week
- 1 celebration meal per week**

Additions in the second half of Consolidation
- 2 servings of fruit every day*
- 2 slices of whole grain bread per day
- 1.5 ounces of hard rind cheese
- 2 servings (cooked cup) of starchy foods every week
- 2 celebration meals per week**

Excluding bananas, grapes, figs, and cherries.
***A Celebration Meal includes 1 appetizer, 1 entrée, 1 dessert and 1 glass of wine. You may only have one serving of each item.*

Use the Dukan Diet consolidation phase to develop your culinary skills with Dukan Cooking!

Protein Thursday and weekly physical activity

Protein Thursday or PP Thursday, is your insurance policy for maintaining your True Weight. Do not skip this rule or you may experience rebound weight gain. Also make sure maintain physical activity – take a brisk walk for 25 minutes daily.

The Dukan Diet Consolidation phase is one of the most important of the 4 phases, which will help you maintain your True Weight permanently.

Dukan Diet Stabilisation Phase

Pierre Dukan firmly believes that defeat on the global weight loss front is largely due to the absence of weight stabilisation in diets. This is why the Dukan Diet therefore attributes as much importance to maintaining a dieter's True Weight through a stabilisation phase as it does to losing weight. Our programme provides every member with adequate support through this phase in the form of stabilisation coaching.

Permanent, life-long stabilisation

This often neglected component of dieting is central in the Dukan Diet. We are committed to extending the programme for successful members, for a nominal fee, regardless of any ups and downs and even if they regain some or all of the weight they lost. Permanent stabilisation coaching costs the same no matter how long you need monitoring, updates and regular assessments.

The phase incorporates 3 simple, practical but non-negotiable steps to help you gradually return to a varied, balanced diet:

1. Eat 3 tablespoons of oat bran everyday.
2. One PP day per week – Pure Protein Thursday.
3. Take the stairs, not the lift.

Stabilisation coaching

After your True Weight has been consolidated, you can decide to continue the coaching programme through the stabilisation phase. Daily monitoring helps you diversify your diet while ensuring a continual balance between energy intake and expenditure. Many people don't succeed at their diet because old, ingrained habits can resurface. In theory, during stabilisation nothing is off-limits and you can eat what you like. In practice, this freedom needs to be managed to prevent weight regain.

The Dukan Diet is a comprehensive diet program with 4 phases: 2 phases to for weight loss and 2 phases to keep your True Weight forever. The completion of these 4 phases is essential. The third and fourth phases of the Dukan Diet, Consolidation and Stabilisation, help you maintain your weight and keep it off for life.Weight loss results may vary.

Cooking the Dukan way

At lunchtime, many people want "good, fast, and a variety." Cooking a meal that meets these criteria is not easy, especially when you're dieting. Here are some Dukan Diet cooking ideas that will make it easier:

1. Use as many of the "100 allowed foods" – lean proteins, adding non-starchy vegetables on PV days.

Consider the seasonality of the 100 allowed foods to receive their maximum nutritional benefits. Choose plain frozen vegetables and you can you save preparation and cooking time. Important: do not forget your daily dose of oat bran which is the basis for the preparation for the Dukan galette (pancake). Do not forget that wheat bran will help you prepare Dukan meals and baked goods. You can prepare some delicious muffins: Remember to beat the egg whites until stiff to create a volume and a fluffy texture.

2. Choose tolerated food items wisely because of their carbohydrate and fat content.

Starting from the Cruise phase, you can have up to 2 tolerated items a day. You can use them to make recipes more tasty. For example, as a substitute for flour you can use cornstarch to make a creamy sauce.

3. Cook without fat:

Marinate your meat, fish and poultry to tenderise them before grilling: use lemon, soy sauce, salt, freshly grated ginger, etc... Use non-stick pans, silicone molds for baking the muffins and cakes, parchment paper for tarts, pies and cookies and bake in foil dishes. Use a steamer and microwave your meals.

4. Counteract the lack of fats with a variety of seasonings.

Think outside the box; let your taste buds discover new flavours: Add spices, herbs, condiments (onions, garlic, shallots, Dijon mustard, etc...) to give a new dimension to your meals, especially during Pure Protein days. Try new combinations: white fish and vanilla, chicken and cinnamon, shrimp and ginger, etc.

5. Revisit classic recipes and make them Dukan-friendly by replacing the ingredients with equivalent approved Dukan foods.

Replace white flour with oat bran, cornstarch, fat-free powdered milk, Agar-agar, or konjac powder. Replace pasta with shirataki noodles and use seasonal vegetables instead of potatoes, low fat cheese instead of regular cheese, skim milk instead of cream, or use silken tofu or fat-free cheese. Here is an example: make tuna salad by replacing butter and cream with fat-free plain Greek yogurt and add any spices or herbs (dill, peppercorns, shallots.)

Dukan Diet Food List

There are about 100 nutritious foods that you can choose from to satisfy your hunger during the 4 phases of the Dukan diet. In the first phase you will focus on eating protein-rich foods only, then you'll combine them with vegetables.

The Dukan diet is a low-carb, low-fat, high-protein diet. Let's see what are those foods that can help lose weight fast:

Lean meat

Beef tenderloin, Filet mignon – Buffalo – Extra-lean ham – Extra-lean Kosher beef hot dogs – Lean center-cut pork chops - Lean slices of roast beef - Pork tenderloin, pork loin roast – Reduced-fat bacon, soy bacon- Steak: flank, sirloin, London broil– Veal chops – Veal scaloppini - Venison

Poultry

Chicken – Chicken liver – Cornish hen – Fat-free turkey and chicken sausages – Low fat deli slices of chicken or turkey – Ostrich steak - Quail – Turkey - Wild duck

Fish
Arctic char – Catfish – Cod – Flounder – Grouper – Haddock – Halibut and smoked halibut – Herring – Mackerel – Mahi Mahi – Monkfish – Orange roughy – Perch – Red snapper – Salmon or smoked salmon – Sardines, fresh or canned in water – Sea bass – Shark - Sole – Surimi – Swordfish – Tilapia – Trout – Tuna, fresh or canned in water

Shellfish
Clams – Crab – Crawfish, crayfish – Lobster – Mussels – Octopus – Oysters – Scallops – Shrimp - Squid

Vegetarian Proteins
Seitan – Soy foods and veggie burgers – Tempeh - Tofu

Fat-free dairy products
Fat-free cottage cheese, Fat-free cream cheese, Fat-free milk, Fat-free plain Greek style yogurt, Fat-free ricotta, Fat-free sour cream

Eggs
Chicken – Quail – Duck
And Sugar-free gelatin

32 vegetables: starting from the Cruise phase
Artichoke - Asparagus – Bean sprouts - Beet - Broccoli - Brussels sprouts - Cabbage - Carrot - Cauliflower - Celery - Cucumber - Eggplant - Endive - Fennel - Green beans – Kale – Lettuce, arugula, radicchio – Mushrooms

– Okra – Onions, leeks, shallots – Palm Hearts - Peppers – Pumpkin - Radishes – Rhubarb - Spaghetti squash - Squash - Spinach – Tomato – Turnip – Watercress – Zucchini

PART TWO: RECIPES

Oat Bran Muffins

Ingredients
- 6 tablespoons of oat bran
- 2 eggs
- 5 tablespoons of zero/non fat yogurt
- 1 teaspoon of baking powder and cinnamon (I heaped the teaspoon of cinnamon)
- Sweetener to taste - I used 1/4 cup Splenda and a cap full of vanilla

Instructions
1. Mix all the dry ingredients in a bowl.
2. Add the yogurt and eggs and whisk until smooth.
3. Add sweetener and vanilla to taste.
4. Divide the mixture equally between 6 paper muffin cases in a muffin tray.
5. Bake in a preheated oven at 350 degrees F for 15 to 18 minutes.

Goji Berry Muffins

Ingredients
- ¾ cup Oat bran (12 Tbls)
- 6 Tbls Wheat bran
- ¾ cup Goji Berries (12 Tbls)
- 1 cup FF Plain Yogurt
- 6 tsp Baking Powder
- 4 large eggs separated
- 3/4 cup Splenda

• 1 Tbls vanilla flavouring (or use lemon,mango or any other fragrant essence)
• Lemon flavouring is very good as well and I put in a bit more than 1 Tbls.
Instructions
1. Preheat oven to 350
2. Beat ingredients together except for the egg whites. Beat egg whites until fluffy and a bit stiff and fold into the beaten mixture. Immediately put into muffin cups that you have placed cupcake liners but best in silicon muffin tins Bake for 16 mins at 350.
3. It will make 12 muffins Freeze when cool and reheat as needed

Chocolate Pudding/Custard
Ingredients
• 2 cups skim milk (approx. 400ml)
• 3 tbsp cocoa powder (reduced fat - sugar free, I use a 10% fat one) you can also use 2 tbsp of cocoa and 1 tbsp of instant coffee sweetener to taste - I usually use 3-4 tbsp
• 2 tbsp corn flour you can increase or decrease this in order to adjust the texture
• 4 tbsp water pinch of salt
• 1 tsp cinnamon, vanilla or flavoring of your preference
Instructions
1. Warm up the milk in a pot on medium heat and add the cocoa powder while stirring until there are no

lumps. a whisk works best for stirring Add the salt and sweetener and keep stirring.

2. In a small cup/bowl mix the corn flower and the water and then add it to the pot along with the flavoring of your choice.

3. The mix will start to thicken as soon as the corn flour is added so keep stirring under low heat for 2 more minutes to avoid lumps forming. Remove from heat and leave to cool.

4. When the mix has cooled pour to serving bowls and then put in the refrigerator

Peruvian Green Sauce

Ingredients

- 2-3 Cloves of Garlic
- 2 Green Onions
- 1/2 Cup of Fat Free Sour Cream
- 1/2 Bunch of Cilantro
- Chicken Stock (enough to blend)
- Salt, Pepper, Onion Powder, Chili Powder
- Fat Free Plain Yogurt (amount varies)
- Lelluce (optional)

Instructions

1. Chop up all ingredients, season and put enough chicken stock to blend in a blender. Taste to see if additional seasoning is needed.

2. Added yogurt to lighten the heat intensity of the sauce and to make it creamier.

3. Refrigerate for an hour before serving with your favorite protein or vegetables.

Steamed Fish Chinese style
Ingredients:
• 1 whole fish (for best results use non-oily fish like bream)
• ginger, julienned
• spring onion, chopped up
• cherry tomatoes, sliced in 2
• shitaki mushrooms, sliced
Instructions
1. Rub fish with salt and sprinkle pepper. Place fish on dish, slit 3 slits on each side of fish, stuff with ginger and spring onion. Also stuff belly of fish. Add tomatoes, shitaki and rest of spring onion on top.
2. Sprinkle a dash of light soy, a dash of Chinese cooking wine and a few drops of sesame oil.
3. Place in steamer or wok over boiled water (use a metal stand) and cover. Depending on size of fish it should take 10-20 min

Hamburger/Sandwich Buns
Ingredients
• 4 Eggs - separated
• 1/4 tsp Cream of tartar 1.23ml
• 1 Tbsp Splenda 15ml
• 4 oz FF Cream Cheese 112g
• 4 Tbsp Oat bran 60ml

- 2 tsp water 10ml
- 1 tsp White vinegar 5ml
- 1 tsp Onion powder 5ml
- 1 tsp Butter Buds Sprinkles 5ml

Instructions

1. Separate eggs. To the yolks add cream cheese, bran, water, vinegar, onion powder, and Butter Buds; mix together.

2. To the egg whites add the cream of tartar and Splenda. Beat whites on high until stiff. Then with the same beaters, beat the egg yolk mixture until well blended.

3. Pour yolk mix over whites and gently fold together. Spoon onto cookie sheet in piles of how big you want your buns to be. You can use a Silpat on your sheets. Other wise use foil with oil spray. Bake at 300 degrees for 30 minutes.

4. You can add any spices you'd like to make these sweet or savory.

Dukan Bread Loaf

Ingredients

- 8 tbspn oat bran
- 8 tbspn wheat bran
- 4 tbspn wheat germ
- 10 tbspn skim milk powder
- 1 tspn baking powder
- 1 tspn salt
- 2 pkts quick fast yeast (8g per packet)

- 1 tbspn no fat plain yoghurt
- 4 tbspn fromage frais or philidelphia extra light cheese
- 3 eggs
- 4 or 5 tbspn warm water

Instructions

1. Use 2 bowls. In the first bowl mix the yeast, water and philidelphia cream cheese and give a good whisk.

2. Mix all the other ingredients together in a larger bowl.

3. Add the yeast mixture to the other ingredients and whisk well.

4. Pour mixture into a loaf tin (I line mine with baking paper) and cook in a hot oven (200 degrees celcius) for 10 minutes. Reduce temperature to 180 degrees and cook for a further 20 minutes.

Low Carb Muffins

Ingredients:
- 2 cups almond flour (almond meal)
- 2 teaspoons baking powder
- 1/4 teaspoon salt
- 1/2 cup (1 stick) butter, melted
- 4 eggs
- 1/3 cup water
- Sweetener to taste -- about 1/3 cup usually works well -- liquid preferred

Instructions

1) Preheat oven to 350 F

2) Butter a muffin tin. You can really do it with any size, but I'm basing the recipe on a 12-muffin tin.

3) Mix dry ingredients together well.

4) Add wet ingredients and mix thoroughly (You don't want strings of egg white in there and you don't have to worry about "tunnels" when you are using almond meal).

5) Put in muffin tins (about 1/2 to 2/3 full) and bake for about 15 minutes.

Variations: Add 1 cup fresh or frozen blueberries for blueberry muffins. For apricot muffins, take a teaspoon of sugar-free apricot jam on each muffin and push it in slightly (it will sink more during baking).

Chicken tikka masala (modified)

Ingredients

- 1kg thighs and drumsticks skinned 1 onion
- 1 butternut squash 4 cloves garlic
- 1 inch piece ginger 3 green chillies
- 2 tsp gar am masala 1 tsp turmeric
- 1tsp chilli powder 1 tin chopped tomatoes 4/5 tbs f/f natural yogurl

Instructions

1) Dry fry onion and then add chillies. Meanwhile mix Ginger, garlic, dry spices together and rub over chicken to leave for a while.

2) Add chicken portions with dry spices ets to pan and cook on both sides for 10 to 15 mins.

3) Add tomatoes and simmer for another few minutes. Cube Butternut squash and lay half of it in bottom of casserole dish.

4) Put chicken mixture from pan on top and then remaining squash on top and between pieces. Casserole at 180 degrees for about 1 and a half hours. Remove chicken from dish.

5) Pour sauce that's left which will quite mushy butternut squash creating thick sauce into pan, add yogurt and half of coriander bringing up to heat again and pour over chicken on serving plates. Decorate with fresh coriander.

Crock-Pot Yogurt

Ingredients:
- 1/2 gallon milk
- 1 cup plain yogurt with active cultures (check the ingredient list! look for "live" or "active" cultures - there are actually yogurts out there that don't have cultures!)
- 1/2 cup powdered milk (non-instant) if using 2% or lower milk or ultra pasteurized milk

Instructions

1) Pour milk into Crockpot.

2) Cover, turn on high and let the milk heat to almost boiling. The actual temperature is 180F which took about 2 hours.

3) Turn the Crockpot off. Take off the lid and allow the milk to cool to 115F or where you can stick your finger

in and leave it for 10 seconds. Stir it around every once in a while as it is cooling.

4) Take 1 cup of the milk and mix with 1 cup of plain yogurt from the store. If you're using powdered milk, stir in now.

5) Put lid back on, wrap entire Crockpot with a beach or bath towel and set away for 8 - 10 hours. I stuck mine in a warm oven that I had preheated earlier to the lowest setting then shut off. I left the oven light on to attempt to keep the warmth constant. I checked after 11 hours and I had yogurt! The whey (clearish liquid on top) had separated off and underneath was a Crockpot full of yogurt!

Meatballs With Rosemary

Ingredients

- 1 medium onion, chopped
- 750g (1lb 10oz) minced beef
- 2 garlic cloves, crushed
- 1 egg, lightly beaten
- 2 tbsp Chinese plum sauce
- 1 tbsp Worcestershire sauce
- 2 tbsp rosemary, finely chopped
- 1-2 tbsp mint or basil, finely chopped
- Salt and black pepper

Instructions

1) Mix together all the ingredient and then shape into meatballs the size of a walnut.

2) Cook the meatballs, a few at a time, in a saucepan over a medium heat for about five minutes until they are golden-brown on all sides. Allow any fat to drain off on to kitchen paper.

Meringue

Ingredients

- 3 large egg whites
- 1 tablespoon antler salt,
- 5 tablespoons (20 g) skim milk powder
- 8 tablespoons sweetener (stro Suketter in the swedish version)

Instructions

1) Beat egg whites lightly with an electric mixer. Sift the antler salt a pinch at a time and continue whisking until batter is thick.

2) Add the dry milk powder and sweetener little by little.

3) Beat the whites until stiff, so that they become fixed, that one can turn the bowl upside down without it spilling out.

4) Click meringue mixture into 8 large peaks on parchment paper on a plate. Bake at very low heat. 100 degrees Celsius for 1 % to 2 hours. Let it cool.

NOTE: Ensure adequate inventory of Appeal in the kitchen where the smell of ammonia, is quite strong for the first hour.

Eggplant Parmesan

Ingredient

- 2 large eggplants, peeled and sliced into 1/2-inch rounds
- ¼ - ½ cup egg whites
- ¾ - 1 cup Italian breadcrumbs, recipe follows
- 3T Parmesan cheese
- Salt and pepper
- olive oil spray
- 3 cups Quick Marinara Sauce, recipe follows
- 1 cup skim milk or fat free mozzarella cheese, shredded or sliced

Instructions

1) Place parchment paper over 2 large baking sheets. Pour egg whites in a shallow bowl, breadcrumbs in another. Dip each slice of eggplant in egg whites, then breadcrumbs, place on cookie sheet.

2) Spray each side of eggplant with cooking spray, season with salt and pepper and lightly cover tops with Parmesan cheese. I use a microplane so only a very little cheese gets used.

3) Bake slices in a 350 degree oven for 35 minutes.

4) Turn oven heat up to 400. Place 1 cup of sauce on the bottom of a casserole dish. Arrange half the eggplant slices, then half the sauce and half the mozzarella. Repeat and finish with two tablespoons of grated Parmesan. Bake for 20 minutes or until bubbly.

Chicken With Lemon Thyme Mustard Yogurt

Sauce

Ingredient

* 1 lb chicken tenders
* ¼ cup chicken broth
* ½ cup plain fat free greek yogurt
* 2 t Dijon
* 1 T fresh lemon thyme, chopped salt and pepper olive oil spray

Instructions

1) Season chicken with salt and pepper, spray with cooking spray, and saute them in a skillet for 2-3 minutes per side, until done.

2) Remove from skillet and keep warm on a foil-covered plate.

3) Add broth to the pan and cook for 1 minute. Remove from heat, add yogurt, mustard and thyme and serve chicken with the sauce.

DD Pizza

Ingredients for two pizzas

* 2 eggs
* 2 tbsp natural yoghurt
* 4 tbsp oat bran
* 1 tbsp cornflour
* 1 tsp of baking powder
* 2 cooked chicken breast cut into small pieces.
* 3 slices wafer thin ham, roughly shredded 2 tsp of parmesan cheese

• 4 cherry tomatoes
• 2 Babybel light, sliced
• 1 tsp mixed herbs
• 2 tsp of tommy ketchup (reduced salt and sugar one of course!!)
Instructions
1) In a bowl mix the eggs, yoghurt, oat bran, cornflour, baking powder and herbs. Split the mix in half and cook in a frying pan, medium heat for a couple of minutes, then under grill for a couple of mins to firm up.
2) Then turn it over in the pan and cook on a medium heat for about one minute. When both are cooked put onto a baking tray, spread a teaspoon of ketchup on each one and layer on the chicken, ham, tomatoes then the babybel and sprinkle on the parmesan. (You could add a few sliced mushrooms if you wanted)
3) Bake in oven for about twenty minutes on 180 (until cheese is as you like it). This makes 2 thin crust pizzas. If you wanted a deep pan one then just use all the base ingredients for one pizza and half the toppings.

Vanilla Cinnamon Cake
Ingredients
• 1 Egg
• 1 Egg white
• ½ tsp Vanilla
• ¼ tsp Liquid Splenda
• 3 Tbsp Fat free cream cheese
• 1 pk French Vanilla Splenda (for coffee pk)

- 1 Heaping tsp Cinnamon
- 1/2 tsp Baking powder
- 1 Tbsp Ground golden flax meal
- 3 Tbsp Oat bran
- 1 tsp Butter buds

Instructions

1) Beat first five ingredients together until cream cheese is thoroughly mixed. Add remaining ingredients and mix well. Pour half of the mixture into a Pyrex or microwavable 1/2 cup container.

2) Put in microwave on high for about 2 minutes or until top springs back. This make 2 cakes the size of a large cupcake. Or you could microwave it all together.

3) The liquid Splenda has zero carbs. You could use Splenda granules no problem; but that may be 3 carbs. I ground the bran just the slightest bit for this. The flax meal gives it nice texture and is all fiber. The butter buds are not essential; you could add extra cinnamon.

Cheesecake

Ingredients
- 1 tbls Oat Bran Splash of skimmed milk
- 2 tbls Quark
- 2 tbls 0% Total greek yoghurt
- Vanilla extract
- Sweetener to taste

Instructions
1) Moisten the oat bran with the milk and press it into the base of a ramekin dish
2) Mix the rest of the ingredients together, sweeten it and pour into the oatbran base
3) Put it in the fridge for 15 minutes

Chicken kiev

Ingredient
• Chicken breast,
• Extra low fat laughing cow,
• 1/4 teaspoon dried parsley
• 1/4 teaspoon garlic granules,
• Salt and pepper,
• 1 egg
• 2 slices DD bread, crumbed,
• Spray light or similar

Instructions
1) Slice into the chicken breast at the thickest point to make a little pocket, mash the laughing cow cheese with the parsley and garlic until well blended, put it into the 'pocket' close it up with 2 wooden cocktail sticks or tie it with string.
2) Beat the egg, then dip the chicken into it, then dip the chicken into the breadcrumbs, pressing them down lightly all over the chicken, lightly spray the baking tray, put the chicken onto the baking tray cocktail stick side up, lightly spray the chicken with frylight , Bake for 30-35mins at 200C. Delicious hot or cold

Easy Eggplant parmesan

Ingredients

• 1 medium eggplant (aubergine) you can peel them but i prefer mine with peel
• cooking spray
• 3 slices DD bread crumbed
• 1 Tbsp grated Parmesan cheese
• 1 teaspoon garlic powder
• 1 teaspoon dried oregano
• 1 teaspoon dried basil
• 2 egg white(s), lightly beaten sauce
• tin of chopped tomatoes
• ½ teaspoon garlic powder
• ½ teaspoon dried oregano
• ½ teaspoon dried basil
• 1 tablespoon tomato puree
• Salt and pepper
• herbs of your choice for the sauce , i like italian seasoning in it
• ½ tspoon sweetener (it gives the sauce a more rounded flavour,)
• 1 diced onion
• 1 very low fat laughing cow (optional)

Instructions

1) Preheat oven to 350°F. spray a small baking dish with cooking spray; set aside.

2) make up your tomato sauce, put tomatoes , herbs onions into a pan and cook until softened add tomato puree, 1/2 tsp sweetener and season to taste with salt

and pepper, you will probably only need half the sauce for the dish but it keeps for several days in the fridge.

3) Combine bread crumbs, Parmesan cheese and herbs in a medium-size bowl; take a 1/4 of the mixture out to use as topping slice eggplant into 1/2-inch-thick slices. put them in a colander and sprinkle with salt, leave for 20 minutes, then rinse and pat dry with kitchen towels, Dip eggplant first into egg whites and then into bread crumb mixture. Bake eggplant on a nonstick baking sheet until lightly browned, about 20 to 25 minutes, flipping once.

4) Place a layer of eggplant on bottom of prepared baking dish, then add 1/3 of tomato sauce cheese. Repeat until aubergine is all used , top with the last of the bread crumbs, dot with laughing cow cheese, Bake until cheese is melted and sauce is bubbling, about 10 minutes more.

Chicken Parmesan

Ingredients
- 1 egg white
- 3 slices DD bread crumbed
- 1/2 tablespoon grated parmesan cheese,
- 1/2 teaspoon garlic powder
- 1/2 teaspoon dried oregano
- 1/2 teaspoon dried basil
- Tin of chopped tomatoes
- 1 tablespoon tomato puree
- Salt and pepper

- herbs of your choice for the sauce , i like italian seasoning in it
- ½ spoon sweetener (it gives the sauce a more rounded flavour,)
- 1 diced onion,
- 1 very low fat laughing cow (optional)
- Nonstick cooking spray

Instructions

1) Preheat your oven to 400° F and lightly coat a baking dish with nonstick cooking spray.

2) Make up your tomato sauce, put tomatoes , herbs onions into a pan and cook until softened , add tomato puree, 1/2 tsp sweetener and season to taste with salt and pepper, you will probably only need half the sauce for the dish but it keeps for several days in the fridge lightly beat the egg white . In another bowl, combine breadcrumbs, parmesan cheese, garlic powder, oregano, and basil.

3) put aside 1/4 of the breadcrumb mixture for the topping. dip the chicken breast in the egg white and then the breadcrumbs mixture until the chicken is coated on all sides..

4) Place the chicken breast in a baking dish and bake for 10 minutes, turn the chicken breast over and lightly spray the top with nonstick cooking spray.

5) Bake for another 10-12 minutes or until the chicken is lightly browned and not pink in the middle.

6) top the chicken breast with tomato sauce and the last of the breadcrumb mix dot with laughing cow cheese.

7) Bake for another five minutes or until the cheese has melted.

La Soupe Miraculeuse (Miracle Soup) - Pv

Ingredients
- 4 garlic cloves
- 6 large onions
- 1 or 2 tins peeled tomatoes
- 1 large cabbage head
- 6 carrots
- 2 green peppers
- 1 bunch celery
- 3 litres water
- 3 low fat beef cubes) far too many. too salty... use fewer + taste 3 low fat chicken cubes)

Instructions

1) Peel and cut the veggies into equal size pieces. Put them in a soup pot with LOW FAT stock cubes and cover with water. Let them boil for 10 mins, reduce heat and continue cooking until the veggies are tender.

Creamy Chicken And Broccoli Curry

Ingredients
- 1 ½ lbs chicken tenders
- 1 onion, chopped
- 1 ½ t curry powder, any that you like
- 1 ½ cups chicken broth
- 1 ½ cups broccoli, steamed

- ½ cup fat-free sour cream
- 1 t cornstarch, mixed in ¼ cup water
- olive oil spray
- salt and pepper

Instructions

1) Season tenders with salt and pepper, a bit of olive oil spray and brown in a skillet for 3 minutes per side. Transfer chicken to a plate.

2) Add onion to the skillet and a bit of olive oil spray and cook for five minutes. Add broth, cornstarch slurry, curry powder and season with salt and pepper.

3) Cook for another 3-5 minutes or until the sauce has thickened a bit.

4) Return the chicken to the skillet, add the broccoli and heat for 2-3 minutes. Remove from heat and stir in the sour cream.

Cinnamon Sugar Flatbread

Ingredients

- 1 packet of rapid rise active yeast
- ¼ cup warm water
- 1/4 cup of oat bran, ground in a coffee grinder to flour consistency a pinch of salt
- 1/2 t olive oil
- 2 t Splenda, divided
- 1 t cinnamon
- pinch of freshly ground nutmeg

Instructions
1) Activate the yeast in the warm water and whisk until disolved. In a double boiler over simmering water, add yeast to the flour, salt, 1 teaspoon of Splenda, a 1/4 teaspoon of cinnamon and olive oil, slowly, until a very sticky ball of dough forms.
2) Spray a glass bowl with olive oil spray, place the dough in the bowl, cover with a kitchen towel and let rise in a warm place for an hour. The dough will not rise much but it will lose it's stickiness and become much easier to handle.
3) Sprinkle some oat bran on a cutting board and roll out the dough until it's cracker-thin (should be about a 7-inch circle). Cut the dough into 2-inch wide strips. Spray with olive oil spray and sprinkle with Splenda, cinnamon and nutmeg.
4) Place on a pizza stone or cookie sheet and bake at 425 for twelve minutes. Eat hot out of the oven.

Braised Tri-Tip

Ingredients
- 1 3 1/2 lb tri-tip
- 1/2 cup dry white wine
- 1/2 cup Worcestershire sauce
- 1 cup beef broth
- 2 T dry minced onion, i love Penzey's
- 1 t Penzey's garlic powder

Instructions

1) Brown the meat in a large cast-iron pan with a bit of olive oil spray. Place fat side down in the pan and season with the rest of the ingredients. Braise in an oven at 300 for 2-3 hours.

2) Slice and serve with pan juices. If you let the dish rest the sauce will be cool enough to strain. Here's the trick: once the juices are cool, pour into a ziploc baggie. (do this over the sink) Once the fat has settled to the top, cut a tip of the corner of the baggie and let the good juices run into a measuring cup. When you get close to the fat coming out, pull it away toward the sink. Then you can reheat it all and you've skimmed most of the fat off!

Chicken and tarragon soup,

Ingredients
- 1 large chicken breast or (any left over chicken)
- 1/2 diced onion
- 3 teaspoon dried tarragon,
- 1 tablespoon dried skim milk
- 1 tablespoon cornflour (cornstarch) mixed with a little cold water chicken stock cubes and 1 litre of water OR 1 litre stock of your choice

Instructions

1) Cut up the chicken, into smallish pieces, add the onion and tarragon,bring it to the boil, turn down the heat and simmer until the chicken is cooked and the onion is soft, about 15 mins whiz it together with a

hand blender until the chicken has broken up into smaller pieces or shreds, add the milk powder and cornflour, bring back to the boil, cook for 2 minutes to cook the cornflour, adjust seasoning to taste

Au Poivre Sauce
Ingredients
• Splash of skimmed milk
• 1 teaspoon on dijon mustard
• 1/2 teaspoon of crushed peppercorns
• 2 tablespoons of creme fraische or fromage frais
Instructions
1) Heat a little milk in a pan.whisk in mustard and peppercorns. Season well. heat over a low heat, stirring constantly. Remove from the heat (to avoid curdling)
2) Add creme fraische or fromage frais. Once mixed together, return to a low heat and heat gently - pour over steak.

White Sauce
Ingredients
• 125ml (4fl oz) skimmed milk
• 2 egg yolks, beaten
• 1 small pot non-fat yoghurt .
• Salt and pepper
Instructions
1) In a double saucepan, heat the milk until lukewarm the add salt and pepper. Pour a small amount of the

milk over the egg yolks, then incorporate the eggs and milk mixture into the pan.

2) Beat well and add the yoghurt. Heat the sauce through.

3) If serving with fish you can add some chopped gherkin.

Creamy Currry Sauce

Ingredients

• 80 grams fat free fromage frais
• 10 grams mustard of choice
• 1 tea spoon curry powder of choice

Instructions

1) Mixed all ingredients together.

2) Can be served straight away, or put in microwave for 30-60 second to take off chill.

Mock Mayonnaise

Ingredients

• 1 cup cottage cheese, low fat
• 1/4 cup egg substitute, liquid
• 1 tablespoon white vinegar -- or lemon juice
• 2 tablespoons Splenda
• 1/2 teaspoon salt -- optional
• 1/2 teaspoon dry mustard
• 1/2 teaspoon paprika pinch pepper

Instructions

1) Combine all ingredients in blender.

2) Cover and blend on medium speed until smooth, scraping down container with rubber spatula as needed. Store covered in fridge.

Yogurt Marinated Chicken

Ingredients:
- 1 1/2 lbs boneless skinless chicken, cut in 1 inch cubes
- Marinade
- 1 cup plain nonfat greek yogurt
- 2 tablespoons lemon juice
- 2 teaspoons ground cumin
- 2 teaspoons ground red pepper
- 2 teaspoons black pepper
- 1 teaspoon cinnamon
- 1 teaspoon salt
- 1 piece minced ginger (1-inchinch" long)
- 6 bamboo skewers (6-inchinch")

Instructions
1) 1 Soak bamboo skewers in water.
2) 2 Thread chicken on skewers, and marinate (in the refrigerator) for al least an hour.
3) 3 Discard marinade and grill.

Leek, Turkey Bacon And Gruyere Crust-Less Quiche

Ingredients

- 2 medium leeks, white parts only, halved, rinsed well and sliced
- 1/4 inch thick
- 8 slices turkey bacon olive oil spray
- 3/4 cup Gruyere cheese, grated
- 2 T Parmesan cheese, grated
- 3/4 cup 1% milk
- 1 1/2 cups egg substitute 1 t salt,
- 1/2 t pepper Pinch freshly grated nutmeg

Instructions

1) Put leeks in a large skillet with water to cover and a teaspoon salt. Simmer over medium heat until the leeks are tender, between 5 and 6 minutes. Drain and place back in the skillet and brown for a few minutes using a little bit of olive oil spray. Remove the leeks and brown the turkey bacon, until just crisp. Transfer to paper towels to drain.

2) Spray a 9-inch glass or pie pan with olive oil and sprinkle the grated Parmesan evenly on top. Put pan on a baking sheet. Whisk the milk and egg whites together and season with salt, pepper, and nutmeg.

3) Spread half the Gruyere evenly in the pan, crumble the turkey bacon on top; repeat with remaining cheese and leeks. Pour egg mixture over the cheeses and bacon.

4) Bake at 350 until the quiche is just set in the center, about 45 minutes. Serve warm or at room temperature.

Homemade Oat Bran Cereal

- 1 egg white
- 2 tbsp oat bran
- 1 tbsp wheat bran 1 tbsp 0% fat quark
- 1 tbsp sweetener (or less to your preference)
- 1 tsp cinnamon or cocoa, vanilla or the flavoring of your liking. I have used cinnamon and fat reduced cocoa so far. Both delicious.

Instructions

1) Preheat the oven to 180 degrees
2) Mix everything in a bowl and then spread on a baking paper with a spatula to create a thin layer of 3-4 millimeters.
3) Bake in the oven for about 20 mins or a bit more if you want them a bit more crispy and darker.
4) Let it cool for 10-15 mins and then break it to little pieces using your hands.

Creamed Spinach

Ingredients

- 1 Bag of Frozen Chopped Spinach
- 1/2 Cup of Non-Fat Milk
- 1/3 Cup of Sour Cream
- 1 Clove Garlic
- Onion Powder
- Salt and Pepper

CONSOLIDATION –

• 3 slices of cheese that are DD friendly (I used pepperjack cheese) again, you won't be able to eat all of this in one sitting

CRUISE –

• Fat Free Cream Cheese - enough to get the cream like texture you are looking for

Instructions

1. Fill pot with just enough water to dump the frozen spinach into. Cook for about 5 minutes.

2. Drain the spinach and dry well. In the same pot, using some cooking spray, saute a chopped clove of garlic.

3. After browning occurs, add the spinach back into the pot. Add milk, sour cream, onion powder and salt and pepper. 1 minute before serving, add your choice of cheese to the pot.

French Toast With Strawberry Jam And Turkey Sausages (Consolidation)

Ingredients

French Toast

• 2 Slices of Whole Wheat Bread
• 1 Egg
• 1/3 Cup of Non-Fat Milk
• Cinnamon
• Salt

Turkey "Sausages"

• 1/2 lb of Turkey (Makes 4)
• Thyme
• Salt and Pepper Strawberry Jam
• 2 Handfuls of Strawberries (consolidation only allows for 1 serving but you won't be using all the jam in one sitting)
• Sweetener
• 2 Tbsp. of Lemon

Instructions

1. Mix together ground turkey with thyme, salt and pepper. Shape into small patties and "fry" using Pam.
2. While patties are cooking, prepare strawberry jam. Dice strawberries, add sugar, and lemon juice. Put on low heat until it reduces to a jam consistency.
3. Prepare egg mixture with milk, dash of cinnamon and a pinch of salt. Quickly soak your piece of bread and put in pan for about 3 minutes on each side (or until brown).
1. Serve French Toast with the strawberry jam and a dollop of fat free sour cream

Strawberry Yoghurt Cake

Ingredients

• 6tbsp oat bran 6tbsp skimmed milk
• 3tbsp sweetener
• 3tbsp natural yoghurt/strawberry yoghurt
• 3 eggs
• 100g strawberry yoghurt fat free 1tsp baking powder

Instructions

1. Simply mix everything together - it is like a runny batter mix. Line the inside of a loaf tin with baking parchment/paper or even better; pour straight in to a silicon baking tray.

2. Put in a COLD oven, and bake on 180C, Gas 4 for 35 mins. Leave for a while, then turn out and leave to cool. You can change the flavour of the cake by adding different flavoured yogurt and essences. I have seen some people also make muffins with this recipe. If you have a pound shop near you

Crockpot Flank Steak

Ingredients

• 1 pound of flank steak,
• V cup of soy sauce,
• 1 cup of pineapple chunks in their own juice (drain the liquid from the pineapples and save),
• 1 teaspoon of ginger,
• 1 tablespoon of sugar,
• 1 tablespoon of olive oil,
• 2 crushed cloves of garlic,
• 3 tablespoons of cornstarch, and
• 3 tablespoons of water.

Instructions

1. To prepare this slow cooker recipe for flank steak you will need to cut the flank steak into about 1/8 inch slices and put them into the slow cooker.

2. Next, mix soy sauce, pineapple juice, ginger, sugar, oil, and garlic in a bowl. Pour this mixture over the steak. Now, cover the slow cooker and cook on low for 6 hours. Turn the cooker

3. on high after the 6 hours and pour in the pineapple and then stir. Mix together the cornstarch and water in a bowl and add to the slow cooker. Cook on high and stir until the sauce begins to thicken. Most people enjoy this recipe over rice.

4. Cook on medium for around 6 to 8 hours. You can also add your own spices like salt, pepper, garlic salt, or onion powder.

Dukan Diet Loaf of Bread Recipe

Ingredients
- 8 tbspn oat bran
- 8 tbspn wheat bran
- 4 tbspn wheat germ
- 10 tbspn skim milk powder
- 1 tspn baking powder
- 1 tspn salt
- 2 pkts quick fast yeast (8g per packet)
- 1 tbspn no fat plain yoghurt
- 4 tbspn fromage frais or philidelphia extra light cheese
- 3 eggs
- 4 or 5 tbspn warm water

Instructions

1. Use 2 bowls. In the first bowl mix the yeast, water and philidelphia cream cheese and give a good whisk.

2. Mix all the other ingredients together in a larger bowl.

3. Add the yeast mixture to the other ingredients and whisk well.

4. Pour mixture into a loaf tin (I line mine with baking paper) and cook in a hot oven 400 F for 10 minutes. Reduce temperature to 350 F degrees and cook for a further 20 minutes.

Quick chocolate muffins

Ingredients

- 2 egg whites
- 50 ml vanilla yoghurt
- 100 g fromage fraiche
- 1 teaspoon baking powder
- sweetener, cinnamon, vanilla and
- 1 teaspoon cocoa powder
- 4 tablespoon oat bran
- 2 tablespoon wheat bran

Instructions

1. It all blended together and stir well with an electric mixer. Executed in six muffins molds bake 3-4 minutes in microwave ovenput in plastic bag and place in refrigerator. may be frozen

Egg Puff Muffins

Ingredients

- 3 eggs

- 1/2 cup frozen spinach, thawed
- 3/4 cup egg whites
- salt and pepper
- mozzarella shredded cheese
- nitrite free turkey breast, low sodium is preferred

Instructions

1. Preheat your oven to 400F. Spray your muffin tin with nonstick spray, and push one slice of turkey into each muffin hole.

2. Mix eggs, egg whites, spinach, salt and pepper, and distribute evenly in each turkey hole. Then top with a small sprinkle of cheese. Bake for 25-35 mins, depending on how brown you want the muffins. Pop out and enjoy!!

Egg Custard Tart

Ingredients

"Pastry"

- 3 tbls oat bran
- Half a cup of skimmed milk
- Heat the milk in a sauce pan, add the oat bran and cook until thick, leave to cool a little.

Egg Custard.

- 2 eggs
- 1 cup of skimmed milk 1 level tbls sweetener.
- A little grated nutmeg.

Instructions

1. Powder a surface with a little corn flour, work the oat bran mixture into a ball and flatten slightly, Put it into a

oven proof dish or cake tin with sides, with your hands mould the "Pastry" around the tin and bake blind for 10 minutes. Gas mark 6

2. Whisk the eggs, milk, sweetener together and pour into the "pastry".

3. Sprinkle the top with ground nutmeg

4. Bake for 30 to 40 minutes (until the custard is set). This could be eaten as a pudding or breakfast.

Chocolate Pralines

Ingredients

- 1 tbsp coco powder
- 1 egg yolk
- 2 tbsp skimmed milk
- 7 tbsp skimmed milk powder (think this cud be reduced....)
- 3 tbsp sweetener
- 8 drops vanilla essence

Instructions

1. Mix the lot together and using a teaspoon put them onto tin foil - then pass into wee paper cups, or direct onto a plate.

2. Put in fridge to set.

Sweet & Sour Chicken

a. 'Fry' off chicken chunks, mushrooms, onions, peppers (i use a LARGE frying pan)

b. In a mixing bowl mix together - then add to the cooked chicken mix.
• 1 cup of chicken or vegetable stock.
• 1 clove garlic
• 2 TBSP soy sauce
• 3 TBSP reduced sugar ketchup (i reckon u cud get away with passata)
• 3 TBSP sweetener
• 1/4 cup white vinegar
c. In a cup mix 2 TBSP cornflour (tolerated item) with a bit of cold water - stir this into the liquid/chicken mix in your frying pan - continue to stir and the mix should thicken a bit. Leave to bubble away nicely to cook off the vinegar for 5 or so mins. IT SMELLS LUSH.

Steak Pizzaola

Ingredients
• 1 steak for each serving - I used New York Strip
• 1/2 green pepper, 1/2 small onion and 4 or 5 white mushrooms for each steak
• DD friendly tomato sauce
• 1/4 cup shredded fat free mozcrella cheese
For the sauce:
• 1 large can diced tomatoes (28 oz.)
• 1 large can plain tomato sauce (28 oz.)
• 1/2 cup finely dice onion
• 3 cloves minced garlic
• 1/2 tsp dried oregano
• 1/2 tsp dried basil freshly ground pepper to taste

Instructions
1. Mix all sauce ingredients together in medium saucepan, simmer over medium heat for 30 - 40 minutes While the sauce is simmering, slice the peppers, onions and mushrooms and saute them in a pan seasoned with nonstick cooking spray. Saute until veggies are crisp-tender.
2. Heat grill and when the grill is good and hot, sear the steaks on one side, Cook about 7 minutes for medium.
3. Flip the steaks over and place the pepper, onion and mushroom mixture carefully on top. Ladel on about 3/4 cup of tomatoe sauce over the veggies. Sprinkle on the cheese and close the grill cover. Continue grilling about 4-5 more minutes.
4. Carefully remove steaks to a serving dish with a wide spatula.

Regularity Muffins
Ingredients
- 140g (1cup) oat bran
- 35g (1/2 cup) wheat bran
- 40g (1/4 cup) linseed/flaxseed (ground in coffee grinder to release more nutrients, or left whole to reduce calories)
- 1/2 tsp bicarbonate of soda
- 1 tsp baking powder
- 1 pinch salt
- 250ml (1 cup) buttermilk, or sweet milk acidulated with 1 tsp vinegar or lemon juice

Instructions
1. Preheat oven to 200oC / 400oF
2. If you don't have buttermilk on hand, stir vinegar or lemon juice into ordinary milk and set aside to sour while you are preparing the dry ingredients.
3. Weigh or measure oat bran, wheat bran and flaxseed/linseed into a mixing bowl.
4. Rub bicarbonate of soda between palms over the bowl, or sift, to ensure there aren't any clumps which would taste foul.
5. Add baking powder and salt, mix thoroughly. Prepare 8 muffin tins (silicone are easiest to unmould and don't need greasing).
6. Add buttermilk or acidulated milk to dry ingredients, mix thoroughly but quickly. Don't overwork. Speed is of the essence here because the acid in the milk activates the bicarbonate of soda and makes bubbles which lighten the muffins; if you wait too long it will lose this effect. Distribute evenly among 8 muffin tins and bake immediately for 20'.
7. Leave in tin on rack for a few minutes before unmoulding. One muffin is daily oat bran requirement and wheat bran tolerance on Dukan Diet. Keeps for over a week in tupper ware container or plastic bag in fridge, can be reheated in toaster or microwave. If you used whole flaxseed/linseed chew well to break them so you get benefit of some of their omega oil.

Speedy 'Attack-phase' recipes
Chicken With Lemon And Capers
Ingredients
- 3 drops of oil
- 1 red onion, finely chopped
- 800g (1lb 12oz) chicken breasts, cut into thin slices
- Grated zest of 1 lemon
- 1 tbsp small capers, drained and rinsed
- 75ml (2% fl oz) lemon juice
- 5 basil leaves, finely chopped
- Salt and black pepper
Instructions
1. In a nonstick frying pan (oiled and wiped with kitchen paper), pan-fry the onion until it turns golden-brown, then put to one side.
2. Brown the chicken slices in the same pan over a medium heat. Add the onion, lemon zest, capers, lemon juice, basil, salt and black pepper. Serve piping hot.

Cod With Mustard Sauce
Ingredients
- 1 cod fillet
- Salt and black pepper
- 150g (5/ oz) fat-free natural yoghurt
- 1 tbsp mustard Lemon juice (to taste)
- 2 tbsp capers
- 1 bunch of parsley, finely chopped

Instructions

1. Sprinkle some salt over the cod fillet and steam for 8-10 minutes (depending on its thickness).

2. In the meantime, put the yoghurt, mustard, some lemon juice, capers, parsley and black pepper into a saucepan.

3. Warm over a gentle heat and pour over the cooked fish.

Vietnamese Beef

Ingredients

- 400g (14oz) sirloin steak
- 2 tbsp soy sauce
- 1 tbsp oyster sauce
- 1 large piece of ginger, grated
- Black pepper
- 3 drops of oil
- 4 garlic cloves, crushed
- A few coriander leaves, chopped Cut the beef into 1cm (about / in) cubes.

Instructions

1. Mix with the soy sauce, oyster sauce, ginger and black pepper, and leave to marinate for 30 minutes.

2. Then cook with the garlic over a high heat for 10-15 seconds, stirring quickly. Garnish with coriander leaves.

Meatballs With Rosemary

Ingredients

• 1 medium onion, chopped 750g (1lb 10oz) minced beef
• 2 garlic cloves, crushed
• 1 egg, lightly beaten
• 2 tbsp Chinese plum sauce
• 1 tbsp Worcestershire sauce
• 2 tbsp rosemary, finely chopped
• 1-2 tbsp mint or basil, finely chopped
• Salt and black pepper

Instructions

1. Mix together all the ingredient and then shape into meatballs the size of a walnut.

2. Cook the meatballs, a few at a time, in a saucepan over a medium heat for about five minutes until they are golden-brown on all sides. Allow any fat to drain off on to kitchen paper.

Salmon In A Mustard Dill Sauce

Ingredients

• 4 thick pieces of salmon, weighing around 200g (7oz) each
• 2 shallots, chopped
• 1 tbsp mild mustard
• 6 tsp virtually fat-free fromage frais
• Finely chopped dill
• Salt and black pepper

Instructions

1. Put salmon in the freezer for a few minutes so you can cut it into thin 50g (1% oz) slices then fry in a nonstick frying pan for one minute on each side. Remove and keep warm.

2. Brown the shallots in the same frying pan, cover with the mustard and fromage frais and allow to thicken for five minutes over a gentle heat.

3. Return salmon to the pan with dill, salt and pepper for a few seconds, then serve.

Eggs Cocotte

Ingredients

• 12 tsp virtually fat-free fromage frais Tarragon (or chervil), chopped

• 2 slices of smoked salmon (ham or bresaola)

• 6 eggs

• Salt and black pepper

Instructions

1. Put 2 tsp of the fromage frais and a pinch of herbs into each of six ramekin dishes. Add a third of a slice of smoked salmon, cut into fine strips, then one egg and salt and pepper.

2. Place ramekin dishes in a high-sided saucepan filled with boiling water like a bain-marie. Cover and cook for 3-5 minutes over a medium heat.

Smoked Salmon Appetizers

Ingredients

• 300g (10/ oz) virtually fat-free fromage frais
• 60g (2% oz) virtually fat-free quark
• 1 small jar of salmon roe
• Salt and black pepper
• 4 slices of smoked salmon

Instructions

1. Beat together fromage frais and quark. Fold in the salmon roe, salt and pepper.

2. Place a little of this mixture on to each slice of salmon and roll up, securing with a knotted chive or cocktail stick. Eat with mini pancakes.

Ham Appetizers

Ingredients

• 175g (6oz) extra-lean ham, chopped
• 225g (8oz) virtually fat-free quark
• A few chives, finely chopped
• 4 shallots, finely chopped
• Marjoram (or another herb, depending on your taste), finely chopped
• A few drops of Tabasco

Instructions

1. Mix all the ingredients together thoroughly. Roll the mixture into tiny balls and serve.

Vinaigrette Maya

Ingredients
- 1 tbsp Dijon mustard
- 5 tbsp balsamic vinegar
- 1 tsp vegetable oil
- 1 garlic clove
- 7-8 basil leaves, chopped

Instructions
1. Salt and black pepper
2. Shake all the ingredients in an old jar. If you like garlic, leave a clove to marinate in the bottom.

Herb Sauce

Ingredients
Makes 2 portions
- 2 tsp cornflour
- 2 garlic cloves, finely chopped
- 2 shallots, finely chopped
- 2 tbsp virtually fat-free fromage frais
- 3 sprigs of parsley, finely chopped
- 3 sprigs of tarragon, finely chopped
- 4 chives, finely chopped
- Salt and black pepper

Instructions
1. Blend the cornflour in 100ml (3^ fl oz) water and, along with the garlic and shallots, add it to the fromage frais.

2. Heat over a gentle heat for two minutes and add herbs at the very last minute. Season with salt and pepper.

Dukan mayonnaise
Ingredients
- 1 egg yolk
- 1 tbsp Dijon mustard
- Salt and black pepper
- 1 tbsp chopped parsley or chives
- 3 tbsp virtually fat-free fromage frais or quark
Instructions
1. Put the egg yolk in a mixing bowl and combine with the mustard. Season with salt and pepper and add herbs.
2. Gradually mix in the fromage frais or quark, stirring continuously. Keep chilled.

Hollandaise sauce
Ingredients
- 1 egg, separated
- 1 tsp mustard
- 1 tbsp skimmed milk
- 1 tsp lemon juice
- Salt and black pepper

Instructions
1. Put the egg yolk, mustard and milk in a bowl over a pan of simmering water. Whisk vigorously until the sauce thickens without curdling.
2. Remove from the heat while continuing all the time to beat the sauce, and add the lemon juice and black pepper.
3. Beat the egg white until stiff and carefully fold it into sauce.

Savoury Pancakes
Ingredients
• 2 tbsp oat bran
• 1 tbsp virtually fat-free fat fromage frais
• 50g (1% oz) virtually fat-free quark
• 3 eggs, separated Herbs, to taste
• Salt and black pepper
For the filling (choose one):
• 175g (6oz) flaked tuna
• 200g (7oz) smoked salmon
• 150g (5/ oz) extra-lean ham
• 150g (5/ oz) extra-lean chopped meat
Instructions
1. Mix together all ingredients for the pancake except the egg whites, until the mixture is smooth. Add herbs and season with salt and pepper.
2. Mix in the filling with the stiffly beaten egg whites, pour into a warmed frying pan and cook over a medium heat.

3. In the second cruise phase of the diet you can use the basic savoury pancake as a pizza base, then dry-fry a chopped onion, add 500g (1lb 2oz) chopped drained tomatoes, herbs, pepper and salt, and simmer for 10 minutes.

4. Spread tomato mix over the base, scatter over 175g (6oz) canned tuna, 2 tbsp of capers and 6tsp of low-fat cream cheese. Bake at 190c/gas 5 for 25 minutes.

Prawn soup with coriander

Ingredients

- 2 low-salt chicken stock cubes
- 1 cucumber, peeled and thinly sliced
- 2 onions, thinly sliced
- 12 large Mediterranean prawns, shelled but tails left on
- 3 sprigs of parsley, very finely chopped
- 2 sprigs of coriander, very finely chopped
- 1 small chilli, very finely chopped

Instructions

1. Bring 1.5 litres (2% pints) water to the boil in a casserole dish and dissolve the stock cubes.

2. Add the cucumber, onion and prawns. When the stock comes to the boil again, cook for two minutes.

3. Sprinkle the herbs and tiny bits of chilli on top and serve hot.

Chicken with mushrooms

Ingredients
- 600g (1½ lb) button mushrooms
- 1 lemon
- Salt and black pepper
- 1 onion, chopped
- 800g (1lb 12oz) chicken breasts, cut into cubes
- 2 tomatoes, chopped
- 2 garlic cloves, chopped
- 250ml (9fl oz) low-salt chicken stock

Instructions

1. Chop the ends off the mushroom stalks and thinly slice the mushrooms, then sprinkle a few drops of lemon juice over them to prevent them from turning black.

2. Put the mushrooms in a nonstick casserole dish. Season with salt and pepper, cover and cook over a gentle heat until all their water has evaporated. Drain and put to one side.

3. Brown the onion in a casserole dish in a little water. Add the chicken, tomato, mushrooms, garlic, chicken stock, salt and pepper. Cover and cook over a gentle heat for 20 minutes.

Quick gazpacho

Ingredients
- 4 tomatoes 1 red pepper
- 1 green pepper
- 2 cucumbers, peeled, deseeded and cut

• Some mint
• Salt and black pepper
Instructions
1. Poach the tomatoes in boiling water for 30 seconds, then peel and deseed them.
2. Grill the peppers for 10-15 minutes until charred all over. Place in a plastic bag and leave to cool, before peeling away the skin and seeds and cutting into chunks.
3. Blend the tomato, peppers and cucumber together with the mint in a blender. Season and serve chilled.

Mexican steak

Ingredients
• 250g (9oz) minced beef Salt and black pepper
• 2 pinches of Mexican spice mixture
• 3 drops of oil
• 2 medium tomatoes
Instructions
1. Mix together the minced beef, salt, pepper and half the spice mixture and mould into small meatballs. Cook in a frying pan over a high heat.
2. Poach the tomatoes in boiling water for 30 seconds, then peel and finely chop.
3. In another frying pan, cook the tomato with the remaining Mexican spice mixture over a gentle heat until the sauce is smooth, then pour it over the meatballs and serve straight away.

Hungarian minced steak

Ingredients

• 6 small shallots, chopped
• 1 red pepper, deseeded and diced
• 3 drops of oil
• 500g (1lb 2oz) lean (5% fat) minced beef
• 2 tbsp paprika
• 100ml (3% fl oz) tomato passata
• Salt and black pepper
• 1 pinch of cayenne pepper
• ½ lemon
• 85g (3oz) virtually fat-free fromage frais

Instructions

1. Fry the shallots and pepper over a low heat for five minutes.
2. Remove from the frying pan, then cook the minced beef for five minutes over a high heat.
3. Add paprika, tomato passata and fried shallots and pepper. Cook for another five minutes and season with salt, pepper and cayenne pepper. Squeeze the lemon juice into the fromage frais. Stir this into the mince, away from the heat, then warm the sauce without allowing it to boil

Herby chicken roulade

Ingredients

• 1 egg
• 50g (1% oz) pink radishes, chopped
• 2 shallots, chopped

- 50g (1% oz) cucumber, chopped
- 3-4 chives, chopped
- 3 sprigs of parsley, chopped
- 1 pinch of tarragon, chopped
- 250g (9oz) virtually fat-free fromage frais
- Salt and black pepper
- 4 slices of cooked chicken 1 tomato
- 4 cornichons (small gherkins)

Instructions

1. Cook the egg for 10 minutes in boiling water until hard-boiled. Mix the radish with the shallots, cucumber, herbs and fromage frais and season with salt and pepper.

2. Spread this over the chicken slices and roll them up. Serve with half a tomato, half a hard-boiled egg and a couple of gherkins each.

Cheesecake

Ingredients

- 5 tbsp virtually fat-free fromage frais
- 2 tbsp cornflour
- 2 egg yolks
- 2 tbsp lemon juice
- 3 tbsp sweetener
- 5 egg whites

Instructions

1. Beat the fromage frais, cornflour, egg yolks, lemon and sweetener until frothy.

2. Beat egg whites until stiff. Fold into fromage frais mixture and pour into a souffle dish. Microwave on medium power for 12 minutes. Serve cold

Cookie

Ingredients
- 2 eggs, separated
- 1/2 tsp liquid sweetener
- 20 drops of vanilla extract
- 2 tbsp oat bran

Instructions
1. Preheat the oven to 180c/350f/gas 4. Mix the egg yolks, sweetener, vanilla and oat bran.
2. Beat egg whites until very stiff and fold into the bran mixture, then pour into a flat baking tin.
3. Bake for 15 to 20 minutes.

Muffins

Ingredients
- 4 eggs, separated
- 8 tbsp oat bran
- 4 tbsp virtually fat-free fromage frais / tsp sweetener
- Flavouring of your choice (lemon, cinnamon, coffee)

Instructions
1. Preheat the oven to 180c/350f/gas.
2. Beat the egg whites until stiff. Mix the other ingredients, then gently fold in the stiffly beaten whites.

3. Pour into individual muffin cases and bake for 20 to 30 minutes.

Fromage frais gateau

Ingredients

- 125g (4 ½ oz) virtually fat-free fromage frais
- 25g (1oz) cornflour
- 1 tsp yeast
- Grated zest of 1 lemon
- ½ tsp sweetener
- 2 egg yolks 4 egg whites
- 3 drops of oil

Instructions

1. Preheat the oven to 200c/400f/gas 6. Mix together ingredients, bar the egg whites and oil.
2. Fold the stiffly beaten egg whites into this mixture. Pour into oiled cake tin, cook for 30 minutes. Serve chilled.

Orange yoghurt cake

Ingredients

- 3 eggs
- 150g (5/ oz) fat-free natural yoghurt ½ tsp sweetener
- 1 tsp orange extract
- 4 tbsp cornflour
- 2 tsp yeast
- 3 drops of oil

Instructions
1. Preheat the oven to 180c/350f.
2. Beat the eggs with the yoghurt, add the sweetener, orange extract, cornflour and yeast.
3. Pour into an oiled cake tin and bake for 45 minutes

Jalapeno poppers

Ingredients
• Fresh jalapeno peppers (this recipe uses 8 -- 4 servings)
• 2/3 of a cup shredded fat free cheddar
• 1/2 tub of Philadelphia fat free cream cheese
• 2 egg whites
• 2 TBS Oatbran, processed in the food processor for a very fine powder

Instructions
1. Wearing gloves slit each pepper length wise but not all the way in half Remove seeds and ribs (greatly reduces the spicy factor)
2. Mix with an electric mixer the cheeses and one egg white. Form cheese mixture into 8 small logs
3. Stuff cach pepper with a cheese log. Beat remaining egg white until slightly bubbly
4. Roll each pepper in egg white then dredge in oatbran powder
5. Place each "breaded" pepper on a cookie sheet lined with parchment paper (prevents sticking without added fat) Place tray in freezer for 10 minutes (to firm up cheese to help prevent leakage during baking

6. Bake in a preheated 375 degree oven for 20 minutes
Let cool for a few minutes

Oatbran Pancake
Ingredients
- 150g cottage cheese
- 2 eggs
- 6tbs oatbran
- 1/2 tsp baking powder
- 4 tbs splenda
- 1 tsp vanilla
- Good splash of milk.

Instructions
1. Put into a blender.
2. Blend and cook! They are yummy. I measure them out using a 1/4 cup measure and that makes about 8, so enough to last me 4 days!

Spicy Turkey Curry - PP
Ingredients
- About 500 g of turkey breast, chopped into pieces
- Juice of ½ a lemon
- 40-50g grated fresh ginger
- Garlic (2 large cloves, crushed)
- 200 ml 0% fat Greek-style natural yoghurt
- 2 tsp cumin seeds
- 2 tsp coriander seeds
- 10 green cardamom pods

- ½ tsp cayenne pepper
- 1 tsp ground turmeric

Instructions

1. Squeeze the lemon juice into a bowl and stir in the ginger and crushed garlic along with the yoghurt.

2. Put the cumin and coriander seeds into a spice mill or grind to a coarse powder with a pestle and mortar then add to the yogurt mixture. Break open the cardamom pods, discard the green shells and grind the black seeds to a coarse powder. Stir into the yogurt with the cayenne and turmeric.

3. Put the turkey pieces in an oven bag with the marinade and leave in the fridge for a few hours, then bake in the bag for around ½ hour (never really sure of the timing...). The yogurt will separate a little as it's not full- fat - then just drain off the liquid. You could also just put it in a oven tray and cook it that way.

Butternut squash soup

Ingredients

- 1 butternut squash
- 1 onion
- 1 lrg piece of garlic
- 10 cherry toms vegetable stock
- 1 tsp ground cumin
- 1 tsp ground corriander
- 2 tsps crushed chillies
- Salt and pepper

Instructions
1. Fry the onions and garlic until soft
2. Add the butternut squash and toms fry for about 5 mins
3. Add stock and spices stir and simmer for 15 mins.
4. Blend with hand blender until smooth

Creamy Mushroom Chicken

Ingredients
• 4 Chicken Thighs
• Bavarian Spices (or combination of spices you like)
• Garlic
• Fat Free Sour Cream
• Bella Mushrooms (1 pkg)
• Broccoli Florets (1 frozen pkg)
• Salt and Pepper

Instructions
1. De-skin your chicken thighs.
2. Season well with Bavarian spices and garlic. Add a tablespoon of sour cream and coat the chicken well.
3. Lightly spray a pan with Pam and saute the chicken until golden brown. When chicken has cooked on one side, flip and add 2 additional tablespoons of sour cream and the bella mushrooms. Turn heat on low.
4. Prepare the broccoli florets while the chicken is cooking. After about 12 minutes, everything will be ready to serve.

Tofu and crab soup

Ingredients
- 1 pkg. of Firm Tofu
- 4-5 Crab Sticks (Surimi)
- 1 Can of Fat Free/Low Sodium Chicken Broth
- Green Onion/Cilantro to Garnish
- 1 Thai Pepper
- 1/2 Cup of Water
- 1 Egg
- 1 Clove of Garlic
- Vegetables (I used bean sprouts and spinach)

Instructions

1. Mince a clove of garlic and put into a pot. Add broth when browning starts to occur. I added a 1/2 cup of water to dilute the soup a bit as there was a bit more sodium than I would have liked in the broth. Add chopped Thai peppers (or any variety) and bring to a boil.

2. Once boiling, reduce to a simmer. Add the tofu (cut into square blocks) and the crab sticks (cut into about 5 pieces per stick). Allow to cook through.

3. Before serving, mix in an egg (for added protein, you may add more).

4. Garnish with green onions, cilantro, etc. and season with pepper.

Oat Bran Cookies

Ingredients:
- 3 tablespoons of Oatbran

- 1 level teaspoon of baking powder
- 1 whole egg
- 1 tablespoon of sweetener
- 3 rounded tablespoons of fat free yoghurt
- 1 tablespoon of goji berries (rehydrated)
- 1 bottle cap of rum flavouring (the tiny bottles of essence)

Instructions

1. Preheat the oven to gas mark 4
2. Mix all the ingredients together in a bowl, folding in with plenty of air until thick and creamy Spoon about 2 teaspoons of mixture into lightly greased individual pots on a muffin/cupcake tray, this produces nice disk shaped cookies
3. Bake in the middle of the oven until golden, about 10-15 minutes. Cool a little before removing from trays onto a cooling rack

Lemon Sauce (for Chicken or Fish)

Ingredients:

- 1/2 red pepper, finely chopped (optional)
- 2 tablespoons equal sugar
- 1 tablespoon cornstarch
- 2/3 cup water
- 3 green onions, sliced
- 1/4 cup lemon juice
- 1 teaspoon soy sauce
- 1 chicken bouillon cube (or 1 tsp dry granules or 2 tsp liquid concentrate)

• salt and pepper

Instructions

1. Combine lemon juice, sugar, soy sauce, cornstarch, bouillon cube, water, salt and pepper in a small sauce pan.

2. Cook and stir over low heat until sauces comes to a boil and becomes thick.

3. Add red pepper and green onions.

Chocolate mousse

Ingredients

• ½ cup boiling water

• 2 teaspoons powdered gelatine

• 1 tsp vanilla essence

• 2 tablespoons cocoa powder

• 4 eggs, separated

• 1/4 cup Xylitol or other sweetner (more or less according to taste....start with less and taste then add more if needed!!)

Instructions

1. Combine water and gelatine in a jug. Whisk with a fork until gelatine has completely dissolved. Stir in 1 ½ tablespoons cocoa. Set aside to cool for 10 minutes.

2. Using an electric mixer, beat eggwhites in a large bowl until soft peaks form.

3. Add xylitol, 1 tablespoon at a time, beating until meringue is thick and glossy. With mixer on high speed, add egg yolks, 1 at a time, beating well after each addition. Add vanilla essence.

4. Slowly pour gelatine mixture into egg mixture (make sure mixtures are both at the same temperature before you combine them), beating constantly until well combined. Spoon mixture into 4 serving cups. Refrigerate for 4 hours or until set and chilled. Dust with remaining 2 teaspoons cocoa. Serve.

Chicken Tikka Masala

Ingredients

- Low Cal Spray
- 1 large onion, peeled
- 1 fresh green chillies
- 1" piece of ginger, peeled
- 3 garlic cloves, peeled
- ½ tsp red chilli powder
- 1 tsp turmeric
- 2 tsp garam masala
- 1 tbsp sweetner
- 1 tbsp tomato puree (didnt use this as on attack)
- 400g tinned chopped tomatoes (didnt use this as on attack used 8fl oz water instead)
- 4 boneless chicken breasts, cubed
- 10 dried curry leaves
- 4-6 tbsp 0% natural yoghurt
- Handful of fresh coriander leaves, chopped

Instructions

1. Squirt a couple of sprays of low cal into a pan, slice the onion and fry. Meanwhile, deseed and chop the

chilli, chop the ginger and add to the hot pan, crush in the garlic and cook for 2-3 minutes to soften.

2. Add the chilli powder, turmeric, garam masala, curry leaves and sugar and cook for 1-2 minutes. Next, add the tomato puree and chopped tomatoes to the pan and allow them to cook for a further few minutes. (or add the water if on attack) 3. Transfer the sauce to a food processor and blend until smooth.

1. Stir in the yoghurt to the curry along with half the chopped coriande and add pre cooked chicken. Alternatively marinade overnight then cook well when ready to eat.

Green Bean Casserole

Ingredients:

- 1 lb of green beans (probably 4 handfuls, it was a bag)
- 5 mushrooms (or as many as you like)
- 1/4 onion
- 1/4 skimmed milk
- 1 clove garlic
- 1/4 cup of fat free cream cheese
- 1/4 cup of fat free mozzarella
- Salt and pepper to taste

Instructions

1. Boil a pot of water and blanche green beans until al dente.

2. Pam a frying pan and add the chopped onions, garlic and mushrooms until browning occurs.

3. Add the green beans into the onion and mushroom mixture. Reduce the heat to a simmer and add milk, cream cheese and mozzarella. Mix ingredients well until sauce thickens and cheese melts. Season with salt and pepper and serve.

Quick chicken soup

Ingredients
- 1 small raw chicken breast cut up
- 2 chicken oxo cubes
- 1 ½ pints water,
- ¼ chopped onion
- 2 teaspoons cornflour

Instructions

1. Put all ingredients except cornflour in a saucepan bring to the boil and simmer for 10 minutes,

2. Take the meat out and put it into food processor with a little of the liquid, blend until the chicken has broken up very small or shreds, put back into saucepan with rest of the liquid

3. Add 2 tsp cornflour mixed with a little cold water and bring back to the boil to slightly thicken

Chocolate Cheesecake

Ingredients
- 5 eggs
- 8 oz. fat-free cream cheese, softened
- 1 tsp. vanilla

- 2 tbsp. low-fat cocoa powder
- 1/4 c. splenda

Instructions

1. Put the eggs in kitchenaid stand mixer and whipped 'em up on high til they were frothy. Then add the cream cheese and beat it on high for a minute.

2. Add the vanilla, cocoa, and splenda, beat til smooth. Pour into a nonstick pie plate and bake at 350 for a half hour. Some sour cream topping would probably be yummy too,

Cinnamon and Vanilla Pancakes with Cinnamon "Butter"

Ingredients

- 3 tbsp oat bran
- 2 tbsp vanilla yoghurt (I used Onken but Muller also make a similar variety)
- 1 egg
- 1 tsp cinnamon (or less depending on how much you like the stuff)
- 1 tsp sweetner

Instructions

1. Mix all of the ingredients well and fry half of the batter on a medium heat for about 3 minutes on each side.

For the Cinnamon "Butter" Topping

- 2 tbsp Philly extra light
- 1 tsp cinnamon
- 1 tsp sweetner

• Makes enough for 2 pancakes.

Jelly-Mousse

Ingredients

• 2 satchets of sugar free jelly crystals (I used strawberry)

• 1 x 500ml pot of fat free yoghurt.

Instructions

1. Add 1/2 pint of boiling water to the crystals, stir until dissolved.

2. Leave to go cool and then whisk in the yoghurt.

3. Pour into dishes and place in fridge to set. it will make 8 ramekin dishes out of this

Prawns for dinner

Ingredients

• 400g green prawns

• 1 chilli chopped finely

• 2 (or more) garlic cloves chopped finely

• bunch of coriander (preferrably freshly picked) - chopped finely.

Instructions

1. Mix prawns, chilli, garlic & about 2 tablespoons coriander together Warm frying pan and when hot give a quick spray with oil, or use a little oil and wipe out - you know how it is done.

2. Add prawn mix and cook for a couple of minutes then turn prawns over. Cook another couple of minutes, try one (what a hardship) and see if cooked.
3. Remove from heat, tip into large bowl and add rest of coriander and juice of lime or lemon.

Cauliflower muffins

Ingredients:
• 1 cauliflower cooked in water to preferable softness (I like "al dente")
• 1 egg
• 10 tbs of skimmed milk parsley, salt and pepper
Instructions
1. Crush up cooked cauliflower, add cold milk to cool down, then add egg and spices.
2. Bake in the oven until becomes firm.

Alexandrian Cabbage Salad

Ingredients
• 1 large head of cabbage, finely shredded
• 1 sweet red bell pepper, finely sliced
• 1 green bell pepper, finely sliced
• 3 stalks celery, finely sliced
• 3 carrots, julienned
• 1 tsp citric acid OR 1 fresh lemon, juice only
Instructions
1. Slice or julienne all the vegetables using mandolin or food processor.

2. Put in the largest bowl you have. Sprinkle with salt and knead to soften the fibres until it begins to wilt a little and reduce in volume.
3. Add citric acid or lemon juice, mix thoroughly. Store in large tupperware container in the fridge.

Sheek kebabs

Ingredients
• one pack extra lean beef mince approx 500g One onion, peeled 4 or 5 gloves of garlic
• One handfull of fresh corriander (remove all the larger stalks)
• 2 chilli peppers-deseeded or more if you like a bit of a kick some fresh ginger
• (these can all be replaced with a couple of spoonfulls of your favourite curry powder or paste to make it PP friendlier)

Instructions
1. Chuck the onion and herbs/curry powder in a food processor and blitz until chopped very finely.
2. Bung in the mince and process some more until you have a smooth mixture. (I will be the first to confess that this does not look very appitising, but keep going).
3. Get the mixture from the processor and give a final mix using your hands. Divide the mixture into about 10 even sized pieces. You now have the choice of either rolling them out between the palms of your hands until they are cigar shaped or you can leave then as little spicy meatballs (just for you Jo).

4. Put the mix on a plate and bung in the fridge for about 1/2 an hour. Put the oven onto gas 6, after time in the fridge space the kebabs evenly on a foil lined tray and put in the oven on the top shelf for about 20 mins. After 20 mins inspect and pour off the excess fat, there is some even when using extra lean mince, into an old tin can. Turn the kebabs and get them back in the oven for another 10-15 mins.

5. Serve with some leafy salad and a dressing of natural youghurt, mint and some finey chopped fresh corriander, you can add some finely chopped chilli to this if you wish. Enjoy.

Simons burger

- Ingredients
- lean turkey mince - or beef mince
- chopped onions
- crushed chilli (if you want it spicy) - or chopped gherkins
- oat bran (optional)
- egg white to bind
- lettuce
- tomato
- sliced onion
- low fat greek yogurt
- french mustard
- large flat mushrooms
- sliced bell pepper (for the mock 'fries')

Instructions

1) Mix the lean turkey mince with the chopped onions, chilli/gherkins and oat bran (optional)

2) Form the mixture into a burger pattie shape.

3) Use egg white to bind if needed, and transfer to the grill

4) Prepare the salad for the burger topping.

5) You can use low fat greek yogurt and french mustard as a delicious burger sauce

For the 'bun'

Cut off the stalks of two large flat mushrooms. Clean with a damp piece of kitchen towel and put under the grill.

For the 'Fries'

Some yellow bell pepper cut into strips gives you something to eat alongside the burger!

Tiramisu

Ingredients

Biscuit:

- 4 eggs (separate white and yolks)
- 1-2 tablespoons of corn starch
- 2 tablespoons of "flour" made of milled oat bran
- 1 teaspoon of baking powder
- 1 teaspoon of vinegar
- sweetener
- vanilla essence

Instructions
1) Separate the eggs, put the yolks in one bowl with the sweetener (I use liquid), starch, oat bran, baking powder and vanilla essence.
2) Stir well. Beat the egg whites with some vinegar until they are firm.
3) Add yolks, stir, put into a baking tray (baking paper recommended). Bake 20-25 minutes, 180 degrees. Let it cool down, cut into "ladyfingers".

Moroccan chicken tagine
Ingredients
• 1 whole large chicken, cut into 8 pieces (I often just make it with chicken breasts)
• 5 tablespoons water
• 1 large bunch fresh cilantro, chopped
• 1 teaspoon cinnamon
• 1/2 teaspoon saffron
• 2 tablespoons sea salt
• 2 onions, chopped
• 5 cloves garlic, chopped
• 1 teaspoon ground cumin
• 1 teaspoon ground ginger
• 1 teaspoon paprika
• 1 teaspoon turmeric
• A dash of lemon juice

Instructions
Rinse and dry chicken and place onto a clean plate.
1. For the marinade: In a large bowl, mix three tablespoons water, the cilantro, cinnamon, saffron, salt, half the onions, garlic, cumin, ginger, paprika, and turmeric. Mix thoroughly, crush the garlic with your fingers, and add a little water to make a paste.
Roll the chicken pieces into the marinade and leave for at least 10 to 15 minutes.
To cook, place in a casserole dish or slow cooker with the rest of the onions. Simmer on low for 50 minutes to 1 hour. (While chicken is cooking excess juices will bubble up and pool around the edges of the tagine; just carefully ladle the juice out into a bowl. After the chicken is cooked transfer the bowl of juices to a saucepan and cook on high, reducing the liquid for about 5 minutes -- essentially making a gravy -- and serve on top of the chicken.)

Dukan Pumpkin Brownies

Ingredients
- 1 cup oat bran
- ½ cup pumpkin
- 300 grams tofu
- 1/3 cup cocoa (no sugar variety)
- 1/3 cup sweetener (i used sugar twin, brown)
- 1 tsp baking soda
- 1 tsp vanilla extract 1 egg
- Dash of milk

Instructions
1. Mix everything together, and mix well! Cook for 20 minutes at 450 degrees.
2. This makes quite a big tray, and gives us a huge serving when divided by 5 (as there is 10 tbsps of oatbran). It taste absolutely marvelous without icing (as we tried right out of the oven)

Low Carb Pizza

Ingredients:
• Whole cauliflower, or small bag of frozen
• 1 egg, or 1/4 cup egg creations
• Random spices (italian spices)
• Low carb, sugar free tomato sauce (homemade would be good)
• Vegetables (pepper, onion, mushrooms)
• Turkey Pepperoni
• 3/4 cup No Fat Cottage Cheese
Method
1. Boil or steam your Cauliflower. Then 'rice' in food processor or blender. Make sure you've tried to get as much water out of it as possible.
2. Then, add spices to 'riced' cauliflower, and 1 egg or egg creations, and mix up.
3. Spread Cauliflower mixture into casserole dish and mash down until crust like.
4. Bake for 20 minutes at 425 degrees.
5. Pour tomato sauce on to baked 'crust' and top your pizza the way you wish.

6. I used green peppers, mushrooms, and turkey pepperon) (2% fat, zero carbs)

7. Add cottage cheese to top of pizza. Bake your pizza for 15 minutes at 425 degrees.

Oat Bran Porridge (Microwave)

Ingredients

- 1.5 tablespoons of Oat Bran
- 200mls of skimmed milk
- 2 teaspoons of allowed sweetener

Instructions

1. Tip the Oat Bran into a microwaveable dish, add the milk and the sweetener and mix. Microwave of full power for two minutes, stir then microwave for one more minute.

2. Remove from microwave, stir well, allow to cool for a minute or two then enjoy.

Moussaka

Ingredients

- 1/2 lb.minced turkey or beef
- 1 onion, diced
- 1 eggplant, peeled and sliced fairly thinly
- 1/2 can chopped tomatoes , drained
- 4 oz. mushrooms, sliced
- 1/4 cup fresh parsley
- 1 clove garlic, chopped
- 1/2 tblespoon dried oregano

- 1/2 tblespoon dried rosemary
- 1 teaspoon cinnamon
- 1 egg + 1 egg white
- 2 tablespoons fat-free cream cheese i used FF fromage fraise
- 1/4 cup fat-free plain yogurt
- Good shake of nutmeg salt and pepper (to taste)

Instructions

Preheat oven to 350 degrees.

Prepare mixture one:

1. Brown mince with onion in a frying pan sprayed with frylite or similar.
2. Add aubergine, tomatoes, mushrooms, parsley, garlic, oregano, rosemary, cinnamon, salt and pepper.
3. Cook until aubergine is tender (about 20 minutes).

Prepare topping

1. Blend together the eggs, cream cheese, yogurt, nutmeg, and 1/2 t. of salt until smooth.
2. Place meat mixture in a casserole dish.
3. Layer mixture topping onto meat mixture
4. Sprinkle top with cinnamon.
5. Bake in oven for 15-20 minutes until top is set.

Fish Curry

Ingredients

- One or two fish fillets, haddock cod salmon etc all work
- a bay leaf
- four peppercorns

- teaspoon turmeric
- teaspoon sweet paprika
- teaspoon ground coriander/ or half teaspoon whole seeds
- half teaspoon cumin
- half sliced red onion
- half a garlic clove sliced
- half a green chilli sliced
- a slice of lemon

Instructions

1. Place onion on top of a sheet of foil, lightly mopped with a little oil/ soy sauce place fish on top
2. Add all other ingredients on top of fish
3. Close foil over at each of the sides to make a parcel
4. Place in pre heatd oven 200 electric, reduce to 180 and cook for 10-15 min
5. Open foil parcel inhale amazing aroma, and serve wit little greek non fat yoghurt (optional)

Smoked Salmon Dip

Ingredients
- 3 oz. of Smoked Salmon
- 1/2 Cup of Fat Free Cream Cheese
- 3 'Dollops' of Fat Free Sour Cream
- Green Onion
- 1/4 Lemon
- Paprika
- Salt and Pepper

Instructions

1. Combine all of the ingredients well and adjust to your liking. For best taste, refrigerate at least an hour before serving. This goes great with Dukan bread! This recipe makes for about 4 servings (so you'll probably be able to use it as a dip for several days).

New York Cheesecake

Ingredients:
- 600g ff soft cheese, we used some Philadelphia cheese but mainly Quark, at room temperature sweetner to taste
- 3 tbsp cornflour
- 1 ½ tsp finely grated lemon zest, preferably using a Microplane grater
- 1 tsp lemon juice
- 1 tsp vanilla extract
- 3 eggs , room temperature, beaten
- 150g fromage frais

Instructions

1. Beat the soft cheese just until smooth with an electric hand mixer on low speed. Gradually add the sweetner, also on a low speed, then the cornflour without overbeating

2. Scrape the sides of the bowl. Slowly whisk in the lemon zest and juice, the vanilla, then the eggs. Scrape the sides of the bowl, then finally whiskin the fromage frais. The mixture should be smooth and quite runny.

3. Pour the mix into the tin . Jiggle the tin to level the mix and squash surface bubbles with the back of a teaspoon. Bake for 10 mins at 190, then lower the heat to llOC/fan 90C/gas

4. Bake another 25 mins and, if you are using an electric oven, leave the oven door slightly ajar for the first 3 mins. After the 25 mins, shake the tin and there should be a wobble in the centre of the filling. If left until firmer it is more likely to crack later. Turn off the oven, keep the door closed and leave the cake in for 2 hrs. Open the door, loosen the top edges of the cake with a round bladed knife, then leave in the oven to cool gently for another 1 ½ hrs. Cover and place in fridge for 4 or 5 hours

Steak mince and onion pie

Ingredients
- 6tbls oat bran,
- 3tbls wheat bran,
- 2 beaten eggs,
- A pinch of salt.

Instructions

1. Make a well with the flour (ground oat and wheat bran) mix in the eggs, When the pastry is mixed, leave for 30 mins in the fridge.

2. Cook the mince and onion, or what filling you would like, turkey and ham, chicken and mushroom, or just cooked veg. This pastry is not the Mouth watering buttery short crust pastry we all know, but its not bad.

Faux Tater Tots/Baked Fries

Ingredients
- 1 Head Cauliflower
- 1 Egg White
- 2 t White Vinegar
- 1 T Powdered Egg Whites
- 11 Onion Powder
- 11 Kosher Salt
- 2 T Reduce Fat Grated Cheese

Instructions

1. Steam cauliflower until tender. When cool squeeze cauliflower in a cheese cloth to get all water out; place in a food processor and add vinegar and egg white; process until smooth.

2. Stir in the powdered egg whites, onion powder and salt and mix well. Put mixture in a piping bag and pipe out one inch tater tots or long fries. Or you could use a spoon to make shapes you like.

3. Place on a cookie sheet and freeze a couple hours. Put frozen tots in a zip lock bag and add cheese and toss till coated.

4. Bake in 400 degree oven for 10 -12 minutes until golden brown. Turn half way through of even browning. These can be baked right away instead of freezing first, but they're easier to coat with the cheese when frozen.

Dukan Kimchi Jjigae

Ingredients
- 2 cloves of garlic

- One carrot, diced
- 500 grams of beef (lean cut)
- 1 kg of kimchi
- 900 ml Beef broth (low sodium)
- 250 grams of tofu

Instructions

1. First 'fry' up some garlic, carrots and beef (in traditional Jjigae, they use pork)
2. Once beef is cooked, add your Kimchi and cook for 5 minutes or so
3. Add beef broth
4. Add tofu
5. Bring to a boil, and simmer for an hour

Dukan Brownies

Ingredients

- 1 cup oat bran
- 1/3 cup vanilla whey protein
- 1/2 cup pumpkin
- 300 grams tofu
- 1/3 cup cocoa (no sugar variety)
- 1/3 cup sweetener (i used sugar twin, brown)
- 1 tsp baking soda
- 1 tsp vanilla extract
- 1 egg
- Dash of milk

Instructions

1. Mix everything together, and mix well! Cook for 20 minutes at 450 degrees.

2. This makes quite a big tray, and gives us a huge serving when divided by 5 (as there is 10 tbsps of oatbran). It taste absolutely marvelous without icing (as we tried right out of the oven). However, I decided to make a little icing for my second piece, which is still 1 serving!

Icing for two
• 3 tbsps Extra Light Cream Cheese
• 1/2 scoop of vanilla whey protein
• 1 tsp orange extract (for the Jaffa lovers!)

Fromage frais gateau

Ingredients
• 125g (4 ½ oz) virtually fat-free fromage frais
• 25g (1 oz) cornflour
• 1 tsp yeast
• Grated zest of 1 lemon
• Vz tsp sweetener
• 2 egg yolks
• 4 egg whites
• 3 drops of oil

Instructions
1. Preheat the oven to 200c/400f/gas 6. Mix together ingredients, bar the egg whites and oil.
2. Fold the stiffly beaten egg whites into this mixture. Pour into oiled cake tin, cook for 30 minutes. Serve chilled.

Meatballs with rosemary

Ingredients
- 1 medium onion, chopped
- 750g (lib lOoz) minced beef
- 2 garlic cloves, crushed
- 1 egg, lightly beaten
- 2 tbsp Chinese plum sauce
- 1 tbsp Worcestershire sauce
- 2 tbsp rosemary, finely chopped
- 1-2 tbsp mint or basil, finely chopped
- Salt and black pepper

Instructions

1. Mix together all the ingredient and then shape into meatballs the size of a walnut.

2. Cook the meatballs, a few at a time, in a saucepan over a medium heat for about five minutes until they are golden-brown on all sides.

3. Allow any fat to drain off on to kitchen paper.

Veggie Curry

Ingredients
- quorn chicken pieces (you can use chicken if you wish)
- 10 cherry tomatoes or 5 large tomatoes cut into quarters half a large butternut squash cut into cubes (part boil first)
- 1 onion chopped half an aubergine
- 2 gloves of garlic bunch of spinach
- 2 eggs

• 20g of pataks tikka masala paste non DD but only 52kcal/3g carb/4g fat

Instructions

1. Sweat the onions & garlic in a wok.

2. Marinate the chicken in the paste, add to wok.

3. Add tomatoes & aubergine, add half a cup of water, add the part boiled squash and 2 hard boiled eggs cut into quarters, leave to simmer for 10 minutes, add in spinach.

Mussel Ceviche

Ingredients

• Mussels (De-shelled package from the Asian market)

• 1/2 a Red Onion

• 1/2 a Lemon

• Cilantro

• 2 Tomatoes

• 2 Cloves Garlic

• 1/2 a Cucumber

• 1/2 a Jalapeno

• Salt, Pepper, Dried Basil

Instructions

1. Saute mussels until cooked through. Set aside to cool.

2. Cut all ingredients into diced pieces.

3. Season with salt, pepper, dried basil and any other spices you like.

4. Squeeze some fresh lemon juice and mix ingredients well.

5. Chill for a bit and serve.

Pizza Stuffed Peppers

Ingredients
- 1 green pepper
- Cooked Ground Italian Turkey Sausage
- Turkey Pepperoni
- 1 Tomato, pureed
- Cooked, diced onion
- Cooked, minced garlic
- Oregano to taste
- FF mozzarella (or low fat feta is really good too)

Instructions
1. Preheat oven to 350 degrees.
2. Fill bottom of pepper with cooked turkey sausage.
3. Mix tomato, onion, garlic and oregano.
4. Top sausage with 1/2 tomato mixutre.
5. Add pepperoni.
6. Top with tomato mixture and sprinkle with mozzarella cheese. Place stuffed pepper on baking sheet and bake uncovered for 30 minutes.
7. Sausage and pepperoni can be replaced with lean ground beef and/or cooked turkey bacon.

Dukan micro bread with marmite

Ingredients
- 2 Tablespoon Oat bran,
- 1 tablespoon wheat bran,

- 1 egg
- tablespoon quark,
- 0.5 teaspoon baking powder,

Instructions

1. Mix up with a fork put into a shallow 4" square micro dish, cook for 4 minutes in the microwave, let it rest for a minute then slice thinly i got 4 nice slices, and i could eat them without toasting them, i ate them straight away lovely and warm from the oven,mix 1 tablespoon
2. Quark with 1/2 teaspoon marmite until it was well blended together, oh boy! it did the job, delicious, this is definetely going to be a regular favourite, comfort food at its best

Pseudo Jambalaya

Ingredients

- 1 package Shirataki Angel Hair Noodles, drained, cut to rice length
- 1/2 package Turkey Kielbasa, cut into chunks
- 1 chicken breast, cooked Tobasco sauce to taste
- 1 T minced Garlic
- 1 half small onion, diced
- Freshly ground pepper
- Optional: diced tomatoes, green peppers, celery

Instructions

1. Stir fry (in water, or in pan sprayed with fat free cooking spray) garlic, onion, cooked chicken breast, and kielbasa. (Add other vegies at this point if desired.)

2. Add shirataki to pan and stir fry until noodles start to shrink (this changes the texture so they aren't so squishy).
3. Add Tobasco to taste

Baked Eggs in Ham Cups
Ingredients
* 1 egg
* 1 thinly sliced piece of 97% ham or turkey ham
* FF cheese of choice (I use ff Cheddar)
* Vegetables of choice (If PV)
* Salt, pepper and other seasonings as desired
Instructions
1. Preheat oven to 400 degrees F.
2. Line a small ramekin or muffin pan with the piece of ham. Fill with cheese and vegetables (if applicable) and top with egg.
3. Bake in oven for about 10 minutes or until the egg white is hard but the yolk is still soft.
4. To serve, remove from ramekin and serve on a plate

Oriental Salmon with sweet soy and ginger sauce
Ingredients:
* Salmon fillets (as much as you like)
* 3 tbsp soy sauce
* 1 tbsp splenda/other sweetener
* pinch of pepper

• grated ginger

• chopped coriander leaves

• 1 sliced chilli (if you like it spicy)

Instructions

1. Preheat oven to 180C

2. Mix soy sauce, splenda and pepper to form the sweet soy sauce.

3. Place salmon fillets on a big piece of foil. Spoon the sauce all over the fillets on both sides, saving ltbsp for later.

4. Sprinkle the ginger, coriander and chilli on top of the salmon then pour the remaining sauce over this.

5. Gather the edges of the foil and scrunch the edges together to form a closed packet.

6. Place in baking tray in the oven and cook for 20 mins.

Turkey and Vegetable Chili

Ingredients

• 1.5 lbs of Ground Turkey

• 1/2 to 1 Red Onion

• 115 oz Can of Tomato Sauce

• 1 32 oz Can of Diced Tomatoes

• 1 Clove Garlic

• Sour Cream to Garnish

• 1 Can of Pickled Jalapenos and Carrots

• Mixture of Cumin, Cinnamon, Red Chili Pepper, Salt, Pepper

• 1 Green Onion

Instructions
1. Saute ground turkey.
2. While turkey is cooking, dice up your onion, garlic, jalapenos and carrots. Prepare spice mixture.
3. Drain the turkey fat and add your spice mixture. Add some reserved liquid (about 1/4 cup) from the diced tomatoes. Cook for 3 minutes.
4. Add the onions, jalapenos and carrots and cook for 5 minutes.
5. Lastly, add the diced tomatoes and tomato sauce. Simmer for 30 minutes or until sauce has thickened a bit.
6. Serve with a dollop of fat free sour cream and garnish with green onion

Asian Beef

Ingredients
• Beef Steak - into strips and fry off with:
• 3 TSP fresh ginger.
• 2 garlic cloves
• Sliced red pepper, mushrooms, onions
• Bok Choy cabbage
• Pour over 1/4 cup beef stock
• 1 Tbsp Soy sauce
Instructions
1. Simmer and cook through to get the full flavours

Dill Salmon with Cauliflower Puree

Ingredients for Salmon
- Salmon
- Fresh Dill
- Half a Lemon
- Salt, Pepper, Onion Powder (any spices you like)

Ingredients for Cauliflower Puree
- Cauliflower
- Skimmed Milk
- Non-Fat Sour Cream
- Garlic

Instructions

1. Squeeze some lemon juice (half a lemon) on the salmon and sprinkle salt, pepper and onion powder on it. For this recipe, I used fresh dill, placing a bed of dill for the salmon to rest on as well on top.
2. Place it in the broiler until salmon becomes slightly opaque (approximately 10 minutes).
3. For the cauliflower puree, boil two cups worth (or one store bought frozen bag) until just tender.
4. Place in blender (I used a Magic Bullet) with some reserved liquid, salt, pepper, a little garlic, a dash of skimmed milk and non-fat sour cream. Blend until you are happy with the consistency.
5. Plate and garnish with some more fresh dill.

www.ingramcontent.com/pod-product-compliance
Lightning Source LLC
Chambersburg PA
CBHW071228240726
48654CB00009B/963